DEMENTIA
HELP GUIDE - VOL. 1

WHAT IS DEMENTIA AND ITS AFFECT ON THE MIND?

WARREN A. PATTON

Copyright © 2024 Warren A. Patton.

All rights reserved. No part of this book may be reproduced, stored, or transmitted by any means—whether auditory, graphic, mechanical, or electronic—without written permission of both publisher and author, except in the case of brief excerpts used in critical articles and reviews. Unauthorized reproduction of any part of this work is illegal and is punishable by law.

ISBN: 979-8-89419-419-6 (sc)
ISBN: 979-8-89419-420-2 (hc)
ISBN: 979-8-89419-421-9 (e)

Because of the dynamic nature of the Internet, any web addresses or links contained in this book may have changed since publication and may no longer be valid. The views expressed in this work are solely those of the author and do not necessarily reflect the views of the publisher, and the publisher hereby disclaims any responsibility for them.

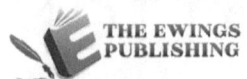

One Galleria Blvd., Suite 1900, Metairie, LA 70001
(504) 702-6708

I dedicate this book to my mother, Adriana U. Patton, an 89 year-old great grandmother who is not only my mom but also my best friend! Many people are not able to say that! She has exhibited early signs of Alzheimer's as well as I. Yes, I said it! I am concerned about my increasing memory loss as well! I also include in my dedication my late Uncle Navarro A. Rhodes who spent most of his adult life a victim of Dementia. May he rest in peace!

"I don't fear death as much as I fear getting old having lost my memory and of not being able to remember the most memorable moments of my life, and of the good times I've shared with friends and family! I can only imagine how frustrated I will become if that happens. But, as long as I am able to remember the Lord, I should be alright! If I do become a victim of Dementia, I will face it with the bravery that I've faced ever other thing in my life!"

—Warren A. Patton

CONTENTS

Preface ix
Acknowledgement xi

I—Part One

1. What is Dementia? What are the Symptoms? 3
2. What are some factors that increase your risks of Dementia? Is it hereditary? 8
3. What are some of the early signs of Dementia? 10
4. I can't remember your name but I recognize your face! 13
5. Self-denial is not the answer! Seek a medical diagnosis! 15
6. FDA-approved medications to treat Alzheimer's/Dementia 17
7. How beneficial are vitamins and supplements? 19
8. Dealing with the frustration of Dementia 22
9. Living with a family member with Dementia 24
10. Senior's stimulate your mind to stay sharp! 26
11. Is there a cure for Dementia? 28
12. Some tips for living your best life with Dementia 29
13. I feel your pain! I too suffer memory loss! 31
14. Resources/References 36
15. Conclusion 41

PREFACE

When I sat down to write this book, I wrote it from the perspective of being a concerned family member, friend and associate, of so many members of our society that suffer from **Dementia** or its symptoms.. Although, I currently don't have it; who is to say that I won't in the future? Can any of you guarantee that you won't be its victim?

Understand that I am not a doctor with a bunch of technical knowledge or high-tech jargon on the subject of **Dementia, brain disorders** and **cognitive decline**, nor am I a manufacturer of supplements that **may or may not** be of benefit in the battle against them. What it is that I'm on your side - that of a concerned citizen, an everyday Joe, with a thirst for knowledge on the subject. I am sure that you have a multitude of questions about **Dementia** and how it effects us! In this book, I will attempt to answer some of the main ones below:

1. What is **Dementia**?
2. What are the **risks** of getting it and is it hereditary?
3. What are **FDA** approved medications to treat it?
4. Is it a communicable disease I could catch?
5. Is there a cure for **Dementia**?

My goal is to gain as much information on **Dementia** as possible and share it with others. This book is intended to serve as a **guide**, a **beacon of light**, a **point of reference**, and an **easy read** for those of you who may be exhibiting early signs of Dementia, have the illness or have friends or family members that do.

My sole purpose of writing this book is that I feel the pain of those suffering from memory loss because I see the signs every day, in my mom, and personally know what it feels like to rack my brain trying to remember significant events in my life - things that I should remember. Understand that I feel your pain and hope that this book will be of benefit to you as you fight the good fight of learning how to cope and deal with **Dementia** and its effects! Be of good cheer knowing that you are not alone! I also share your journey!

I hope this book will provide courage to those who are hiding their symptoms from family and friends. The kind of courage that will allow you to humble yourselves enough to seek help! I thank the Lord for giving me the courage to write this book and leave behind something that I feel will help my fellow man! **Amen!**

ACKNOWLEDGEMENT

I would like to take this opportunity to acknowledge the hundreds of people who have played a import part of in my life from my grade school, Ernie Pyle Elementary; junior high school Tolleston High; high school, Gary West Side High; hometown, Gary, IN; colleges attend: South Carolina State College, Orangeburg, SC; Chaminade University, Honolulu, HI; Troy State University, Troy, AL, Southwest Region; U.S. Navy duty assignments: Naval Training Center (Boot Camp), Great Lakes, IL; Navy School of Broadcast Journalism, DINFOS, Fort Benjamin Harrison, IN; Pre-commissioning crew, USS Cimarron (AO-177), San Diego, CA; Commander Naval Base, Pearl Harbor, HI; Commander Naval Station, Treasure Island, CA; Navy Recruiting District, San Francisco, CA; Officer Candidate School (OCS), Newport, RI; Navy Recruiting Orientation Unit (NORU), Pensacola, Fl; and Navy Recruiting Area EIGHT (NAVCRUIT Area EIGHT). I would also acknowledge the unnamed friends, family and associates, who have been with me through the good and the bad. You know who you are, thus the reason for me to protect your right to privacy. I love you all and want to acknowledge you while I am still able to remember! Be blessed!

I
PART ONE

1

WHAT IS DEMENTIA? WHAT ARE THE SYMPTOMS?

The **World Health Organization (WHO)** states that,**"Dementia** is an **umbrella term** for several diseases affecting memory, other cognitive abilities and behavior that interfere significantly with a person's ability to maintain their activities of daily living. Although age is the strongest known risk for dementia, it is **not** a normal part of aging." - **www.who.int - 2023**

The **Alzheimer's Association** goes on to state,"Dementia is **not** a single disease, it's an overall term – like heart disease - that covers a wide range of specific medical conditions, including Alzheimer's disease. Disorders grouped under the general term **"Dementia"** are caused by abnormal brain changes. These changes trigger a decline in thinking skills, such as cognitive abilities, severe enough to impair daily life and independent function. They also affect behavior, feelings, and relationships." - **www.alz.org - 2023**

According to **American Seniors Communities (ASC)**, "When people think of **Dementia**, it's common to think of it as a mental illness due to the effects the condition has on the brain. However, there are distinctions that should be made between **Dementia** and mental illness in order to properly diagnose the individual. While **Dementia** does affect mental health, it **is NOT a mental illness, but a disorder of the brain** that causes memory loss and trouble with communicating. Proper diagnosis of mental illness or **Dementia** in the elderly is vital in order to ensure that proper treatment is provided as soon as possible. Misdiagnosis of mental illness in seniors can occur easily since symptom are so similar to **Dementia**, like confusion and erratic behavior" – www.asccare - **Feb 19, 2015**

As defined by the **Food and Drug Administration (FDA)** - "**Dementia** is a serious and debilitating neurological condition characterized by progressive decline in one or more cognitive domains in the brain. **Dementia** can seriously impair an individual's ability to function independently. Many people living with dementia require permanent at-home or residential care. **Azheimer's Disease is the most common cause of Dementia.** Alzheimer's disease is an irreversible, progressive brain disorder affecting more than 6.5 million Americans. Patients with **Dementia** often have behavioral and psychological disturbances. Agitation is among the most persistent, complex, stressful, and costly aspects of care among patients with behavioral and psychological symptoms of dementia." - www.fda.org -

May 11, 2023

The **Merriam-Webster dictionary** defines **Dementia** as: "…a usually progressive condition (such as Alzheimer's disease) marked by the development of multiple cognitive deficits (such as memory impairment, aphasia, and the inability to plan and initiate complex behavior.)" – www.merriam-webster.com - May 26, 2023

The **Centers for Disease Control and Prevention (CDC)** lists the most common types of **Dementia** as:

- **Alzheimer's disease:** The most common cause of dementia, accounting for 60 to 80 percent of cases caused by specific changes in the brain. The trademark symptom is trouble remembering recent events, such as a conversion that occurred minutes or hours ago.

- **Vascular Dementia:** With about 10 percent of dementia cases linked to stroke or other issues with blood flow to the brain. Diabetes, high blood pressure and high cholesterol are also risk factors. ….The disease progresses in a stepwise fashion, meaning symptoms will suddenly get worse as the individual gets more strokes or mini-strokes.

- **Lewy Body Dementia:** Along with more typical symptoms like memory loss, people with this form of Dementia may have movement or balance problems like stiffness or trembling. Many people also experience changes in alertness, including daytime sleepiness.

- **Fronto-temporal Dementia:** This type of Dementia most often leads to changes in personality and behavior because of the part of the brain it affects. People with this condition may embarrass themselves or behave inappropriately. For instance, responsibilities at home or work. There may also be problems with language skills like speaking or understanding.

Note: The information above was obtained from www.cdc.gov-/aging/dementia - dated April 5, 2019

According to **Open Systems Healthcare, (OSH)** "Many early signs of Dementia go unnoticed because symptoms are often accredited to normal aging. However, early diagnosis is ideal, so it is important to be aware of the early signs. If your-loved one has experienced any of the following symptoms, it is a good time to schedule a consultation with your doctor. Symptoms include memory loss, inability to reason, problems with language or communication, impaired vision, and lack of attention or focus.

"Dementia is caused by damage to brain cells, impairing a brain region's ability to function. The specific region of the brain that is impaired depends on the type of Dementia. The most common type is Alzheimer's Dementia, followed by vascular Dementia. There are also types of Dementia that are more treatable, such as Dementia due to Vitamin deficiencies or depression. Alzheimers is a progressive disease and the most common cause of Dementia. This means that symptoms of Dementia worsen over time, as brain cells continually degrade. The **symptoms of Alzheimer's** may include memory loss, disorientation, difficulty learning, mood changes, and confusion about time. While there is no known cure for Alzheimer's, researchers are working to find ways to better treat the disease." - www.opensystemshealthcare.com - Sept 6, 2019

How is **Dementia** different from **Alzheimer's** and which one comes first? "Alzheimer's disease starts in the brain many years before symptoms start to show. Early symptoms are mild and don't stop someone from doing their normal everyday activities. It's only later that symptoms become severe enough to be called **Dementia**." – **Mayo Clinic** - www.mayoclinic.org - October 12, 2021

WHAT IS DEMENTIA? WHAT ARE THE SYMPTOMS?

"**Dementia** is a group of symptoms of which Alzheimer's is one. It is progressive, which means symptoms may be relatively mild at first, but get worse over time. **Alzheimer's** disease is the most common cause of Dementia. Eventually Azheimer's disease causes so much damage to the brain that the person develops Dementia." – **www.alzheimers.org.uk - August 3, 2023**

2

WHAT ARE SOME FACTORS THAT INCREASE YOUR RISKS OF DEMENTIA? IS IT HEREDITARY?

According to the CDC there are factors that increase your risk for Dementia such as "Age; Family History; Race/Ethnicity; Poor heart health and Traumatic brain injury."

Basically stated, "The strongest known risk factor for Dementia is increasing age, with most cases affecting those of 65 years and older. Those individuals who have parents or siblings with Dementia are more likely to develop Dementia themselves. Race/ethnicity is also a factor with, "Older African Americans are twice more likely to have Dementia than whites, Hispanics 1.5 times more likely to have Dementia than whites."

"Poor heart health, high cholesterol, and smoking increase the risk of Dementia if not treated properly. Traumatic brain injury or any type of injury to the head can increase the risk of Dementia, especially if they are severe or occur repeatedly." – www.cdc.org -

WHAT ARE SOME FACTORS THAT INCREASE YOUR RISKS OF DEMENTIA? IS IT HEREDITARY?

April 5, 2019

When thinking about all these factors, I think about the risk that professional boxers, wrestlers, mixed-martial artists, take each time they get in the ring. What about repeated concussions received by football players, young or old?

The CDC goes on to say that Dementia is NOT a part of normal aging and that, "many older adults live their entire lives without developing Dementia, and that normal aging may include weakening muscles and bones, stiffening of arteries and vessels, and some age-related memory changes that may show up as:

Occasionally misplacing our car keys
Struggling to find a word but remembering it later
Forgetting the name of an acquaintance or family member
Forgetting the most recent events

The National Center for Complementary and Integrative Health (NCCIH) states that, "Concerns about forgetfulness and whether it is the first sign of Alzheimer's disease are common, particularly among older patients. What science says about dietary supplements and Cognitive Function, Dementia, and Alzheimer's disease, is that although a few trials of natural products for the prevention of cognitive decline or Dementia have shown some modest effects, direct evidence is lacking. In addition, research on some mind and body practices, such as music therapy and mental imagery, which have shown promise in treating some symptoms related to Dementia, as well as alleviating stress among caregivers, is ongoing." – www.nccih.gov - July 2022

3

WHAT ARE SOME OF THE EARLY SIGNS OF DEMENTIA?

"What is the earliest symptom of **Dementia**? The answer: Difficulties with memory! Whether it be with yourself, friends or family members: For example, a person may not recall events or may keep losing items (such as keys and glasses) around the house. Memory loss is often the first and main symptom in early Alzheimer's disease."—**www.betterhealth.vic.gov.au** - page review May 31, 2014

If you or your loved-ones exhibit several of these 10 symptoms of Dementia, consult your Doctor for a complete evaluation:

- **Memory loss:** It's quite normal for most of us to occasionally forget appointments and remember them later. However, a person with **Dementia** may forget things more often or not remember them at all.

- **Language problems:** Most of us have trouble finding the right word to use sometimes, but a person with **Dementia**

WHAT ARE SOME OF THE EARLY SIGNS OF DEMENTIA?

may forget simple words or substitute inappropriate words, making sentences difficult to understand. They may also have trouble understanding others.

- **Mood, personality or behavior changes:** Everyone of us has been sad or moody at some point or another. But, someone with Dementia can have rapid mood swings, for no apparent reason. They may become confused, suspicious, paranoid or withdrawn. Some can become uninhibited or more outgoing.

- **Loss of initiative:** It is normal to tire of some activities. However, Dementia may cause a person to lose interest in an activity they previously enjoyed and require cues prompting them to become involved.

- **Poor spatial skills:** A person with **Dementia** may have difficulty judging distance or direction while driving a car.

- **Misplacing thing:** Each of us at some point in time has temporarily misplaced a wallet or keys. However, a person with **Dementia** may not know what the keys are for.

- **Disorientation:** A person with **Dementia** may get disoriented and have difficulty finding their way to a familiar place or feel confused about where they are, or think they are back in some past time in their life.

- **Poor judgment:** Many activities in our lives require good judg-ment. But, when this ability is affected by **Dementia**, the person may have difficulty making appropriate decisions, such as what to wear in cold weather.

- **Changes in abstract thinking:** Anyone can have difficulty man-aging finances, but a person with **Dementia** may have trouble knowing what the numbers mean or what to do with them.

- **Difficulty with tasks:** People may get distracted when serving a meal and forget part of it. But, a person with **Dementia** may have trouble with all the steps in preparing the meal.

What increases the risk for Dementia?

- **Age:**
  The strongest known risk factor for **Dementia** is increasing age, with most cases affecting those of 65 years and older

- **Family history:**
  Those who have parents or siblings with **Dementia** are more likely to develop dementia themselves.

- **Race/ethnicity:**
  Older African Americans are twice more likely to have **Dementia** than whites. Hispanics are 1.5 times more likely to have **Dementia** than whites.

- **Poor heart health:**
  High blood pressure, high cholesterol, and smoking increase the risk of **Dementia** if not treated properly.

- **Traumatic brain injury:**
  Head injuries can increase the risk of **Dementia**, especially if they are severe or occur repeatedly. – **www.betterhealth. vic.gov.au** - page review May 31, 2014

4

I CAN'T REMEMBER YOUR NAME BUT I RECOGNIZE YOUR FACE!

If you want to be embarrassed, tell someone that you can't remember their name but you recognize their face. This is probably normal for those of us over the age of 65, but the truth is I can't remember the names of most of the females that I dated while attending South Carolina State College in Orangeburg, SC. I would need to get my hands on a yearbook from that period of time and look at some pictures in order to remember them. Has this happened to you?

If you look at someone and have an overwhelming feeling that you should know this person, but can't remember who they are or where you know them from, you may possibly be experiencing early signs of Dementia. In which case, don't hesitate to do something about it.

Don't let your pride or ego prevent you from seeking medical advice. The earlier that you do something about it, the better off you will be! You may just be experiencing a false alarm and normal signals that come with aging. Remember, there are some of us who live to be 100, with still control of all our faculties. My uncle Francisco, before he died, was in an assisted living facility and was sharp as a tack with regard to his memory! How did he do it? Working crossword puzzles daily. In fact, I used to take a new puzzle book with me every time I went to visit him or pick him up to spend time with him.

Should you actually be worried about forgetting names? Well, according to **Hartford Healthcare Geriatrician, Taimur Habib, MD**, "Not being able to recall a word or name is certainly annoying. But usually, that's all it is! For most people, it's not a sign of something worse." – **www.health.harvard.edu - Aug 12, 2022**

But, on the other hand there is a medical condition for forgetting names called: **Primary Progressive Aphasia (PPA)**, which is "…a rare type of **Dementia**, where language is heavily affected. As it's primary progressive condition, the symptoms get worse over time. Usually, the first problem people with PPA notice is difficulty finding the right word or remembering somebody's name," according to the **Mayoclinic.org, www.mayoclinic.org - page review April 1, 2023.**

5

SELF-DENIAL IS NOT THE ANSWER! SEEK A MEDICAL DIAGNOSIS!

"Hey man, I'm alright! There is nothing wrong with my memory. Give me a minute and I'll remember his or her name!" How many of us have been the aforementioned person? Allowing self-denial with regard to our memory, of denying the fact that we just don't remember?

The fact is that when a person denies the onset of **Dementia**, he or she denies themselves the truth, they also negatively affect those around them, who know better!

It's quite normal for people to forget things! Most of us have experienced this type of thing, or may have forgotten where you laid your car keys, wallet, purse, etc., and the frustration that you feel trying to find it. What I have found to be the case is that quite a few Seniors are in self-denial of the fact that they may be experiencing the onset of **Dementia**. The truth is that it is nothing to be ashamed of!

Self-denial is definitely not the answer! Once, I admitted to myself that I might be experiencing some loss of memory. I went online to research everything that I could find on the subject, possible treatments, etc.

If you are worried that this may be happening to you, seek a medical diagnosis. According to the **Center for Disease Control**, "A healthcare provider can perform tests on attention, memory, problem solving and other cognitive abilities to see if there is a cause for concern. A physical exam, blood tests, and brain scans like a CT or MRI can help determine an underlying case." – www.cdc.gov/aging/dementia **page review April 5, 2019**

How do we offer help to someone who denies that they need help? According to **Alzheimers.org.uk**, "It is common for someone living with Dementia to deny that they are experiencing issues with their memory or other aspects of cognition, such as having difficulty holding conversations or carrying out daily living tasks.

"This could be due to denial or lack of insight. Similar to denial, lack of insight means that a person with Dementia is unable to recognize changes in their behavior and personality." – www.alzheimers.org.uk **page review May 23, 2023**

Now the problem is with your family member, friend, or loved one, continuing to deny that something is wrong with them, they may continue to refuse help, stop taking any medications, continue to drive even though they shouldn't, or operate unsafe tools around the house like power-saws, etc., causing danger to themselves or others.

6

FDA-APPROVED MEDICATIONS TO TREAT ALZHEIMER'S/DEMENTIA

My internet search revealed that the **Food and Drug Administration (FDA)** has approved different types of drugs specifically to treat symptoms of Alzeimer's disease, which once it gets worse becomes Dementia. The following drugs which can be self-administered as a pill, time-release capsule, skin patch or syrup, include **three cholinesterase inhibitors** and **Memantine** listed below:

The FDA has approved the following medications:

Donepezil (also known as Aricept), rivastigmine (Exelon) and galantamine (Reminyl) are used to treat the symptoms of mild to moderate Alzheimer's disease. **Donepezil is also used to treat more severe Alzheimer's disease.**

Donepezil (Aricept) - approved to treat all stages of Alzheimer's disease Dementia. It's taken once a day as a pill.

Galantamine (Razadyne) - approved to treat mild to moderate Alzheimer's disease. It's taken as a pill once a day or as an extended-release capsule twice a day.

Rivastigmine (Exelon) - approved for mild to moderate Alzheimer's disease. It's taken as a pill. A skin patch is available that can also be used to treat severe Alzheimer's disease.

Memantine (Namenda) - approved for treatment of **moderate to severe Alzheimer's disease**. It works by regulating the activity of glutamate, a messenger chemical widely involved in brain functions - including learning and memory. It's taken as a pill or syrup;

The **FDA** has also approved a combination of **Donepezil** and **Memantine (Namzaric)**, which is taken as a capsule.

What is the newest FDA-approved drug for dementia?

"Today, the U.S. Food and Drug Administration is announcing the supplemental approval of Rexulti (brexpiprazole) oral tablets for the treatment of agitation associated with dementia due to Alzheimer's disease. This is the first FDA-approved treatment option for this indication." - www.fda.org news release May 11, 2023

7

HOW BENEFICIAL ARE VITAMINS AND SUPPLEMENTS?

With regard to Dementia, there is **no known cure** for it, but there are **multivitamins, vitamins** and **supplements** that may help to fight against the loss of memory and some that may actually help improve memory. Note: None of which are approved by the **Food and Drug Administration (FDA)**.

My research also revealed vitamins and supplements that may be of benefit in the fight against Dementia. It is important to note here that **"...dietary supplements, including multivitamins and vitamins are NOT approved by the U.S. Food and Drug Administration. This also includes cognitive health supplements as well as homeopathic remedies."** – www.fda.org news release May 11, 2023

Here are some highly touted **Brain Supplements** which **may** possibly improve and help slow cognitive decline. Some of which include:

- Huperzine A
- Ginkgo Biloba
- Vitamin B12 and other B vitamins
- Omega-3 fatty acid supplements
- Vitamin E
- Magnesium
- L-theanine
- Curcumin (Turmeric)
- Vitamin D
- Prevagen
- Nuriva
- Bacopa Monnieri

"For **older adults**, taking a daily multivitamin may improve memory and help slow age-related cognitive decline, according to new research from **Columbia University in New York and Brigham, and Women's Hospital/Harvard in Boston, MA**." – www.cbsnews.com news release - May 24, 2023

Personally, **I am not a medical authority on the subject of Dementia**, but I am one of those individuals who believes in doing my homework on the subject, and very willing to try highly recommended products that could possibly help me with my memory. In fact, I currently take memory supplements myself in the hopes that I can improve my memory and delay the onset of memory loss.

The fact is, you can find just about any subject that you want to on the internet and these are some things that I hope may be of help to those suffering from Dementia or those exhibiting symptoms that they want to do something about.

HOW BENEFICIAL ARE VITAMINS AND SUPPLEMENTS?

"Taking Supplements for **Dementia**, many people, including those who are not currently experiencing any signs or symptoms of cognitive decline, **may** benefit from targeted supplementation of essential vita-mins and minerals. While there is currently **no cure for Alzheimer's disease or Dementia**, ensuring that the body has an adequate level of essential nutrients **may** help to ward off disease and improve well-being.". – **www.careforth.com article by Angela Stringfellow, May 17, 2018**

Does anything really improve memory? "Regular exercise boosts the growth of brain cells and the production of neurotransmitters, enhancing memory. A mixture of aerobic and strength exercises is best. If you're not getting enough sleep, you might be harming your cognition and memory. Aim for seven to nine hours each night." – **www.health.harvard.edu review August 12, 2022**

8

DEALING WITH THE FRUSTRATION OF DEMENTIA

Do **Dementia** patients get frustrated? Absolutely? Not being able to remember faces, places, events, etc., is frustrating for everyone whether they have **Dementia** or not!

What is really sad is seeing a family member or friend break down and cry because of not being able to remember you or your name. I'm talking about someone who has known you for most of your life or theirs. I can sympathize with this because there are times that I have felt like crying about forgetting the name of someone that I've known since kindergarten, this even extends to relatives. In most cases, I will pretend to remember them, hoping that someone else present calls out their name. How many of you have this happened too?

Turning age 69 this October 15, 2023, I can identify with all those Seniors over the age of 65, who may be experiencing memory loss or the onset of Alzheimer's, which is one of the precursors of Dementia, especially those individuals who don't have a clue that this may be happening to them.

"The loss of cognitive functions such as reasoning, memory, problem-solving,and judgment. These symptoms may make a person with Dementia feel embarrassed,frustrated, and patronized, causing them to react with meanness and anger," according to **Medical News Today**. - www.medicalnewstoday – Aug 23, 2022

The article goes on to say, "Changes in personality and behavior are common in people with Dementia. These changes may involve angry outbursts and aggressive behaviors such as shouting verbal threats, physical violence, and damaging property. Understanding the reasons for their behavior can help prevent the behaviors from happening again and help caregivers respond and cope better."

The **Alzheimer's Association** lists several tips for Caregivers of **Dementia** to help them respond to angry outbursts and changing behaviors as follows:

- **Try to identify the origin or cause**
- **Distract them**
- **Respond appropriately, using short and simple sentences**
- **Give them space and time**
- **Respond calmly, using a calm tone of voice**
- **Do not take attacks personally**
- **Talk with them with respect, not as children**

9

LIVING WITH A FAMILY MEMBER WITH DEMENTIA

How does a person deal with **Dementia**? How does a family or friends deal with a loved-one who is a victim of disease?

As a person who has **Dementia**, you should "…set realistic goals and focus on what you can do today. Set realistic expectations for yourself and use the skills you have to be successful in dealing with challenging tasks Some tasks may become too difficult for you to complete even with reminder aids. Reduce stress by asking family or friends for help, if needed," says the **Alzheimer's Association** –www.alz.org 2023

Now here is where I absolutely agree with the **Alzheimer's Association** with regard to reminder aids. Because, I know that if I don't write things down on a "To Do List" or a "Tickler List", there is a very good chance that I will not remember important things that need to be done later that day, the next day, or the next week. Forgetting very simple things is stressful for everyone, especially those with **Dementia** or early warning signs of **Alzheimer's**, a precursor of **Dementia**.

When you're dealing with a person with Alzheimer's, or its more advanced stage Dementia, I recommend that you go on the internet and look at some of the videos on Youtube and other social sites that show videos of tips from Caregivers with experience on how to delicately deal with someone with the disease. Here are some of the common tips that some of them shared:

- **Never argue with them**
- **Never remind them about a family member or love-one who died**
- **Never tell them they are wrong about something**
- **Never bring up any subjects that you think may upset them**
- **Never accuse them of anything**
- **Never say anything you think may embarrass them**
- **Never ignore them or give them the silent treatment**

As a loved one of a family with **Dementia** your focus should be on showering that person with as much love and affection as possible, and do everything in your power to see that your loved one has the best quality of life that is within your power to provide. Remember, that could easily be you!

As a **Caregiver** of that person, become a student of the Disease, learning everything that you possibly can about what signs to look for as they progress through the disease, how to care for them, how to relate to them, etc. Every bit of information that you need is readily available to you on the internet.There is no need to go to the Library. If you are not computer literate, get help from a family member or friend with those skills.

10

SENIOR'S STIMULATE YOUR MIND TO STAY SHARP!

One of the best recommendations that I can make for someone who is getting on in age, and thinks they are experiencing early signs of **Dementia**, is to stimulate your mind as much as possible. I'm talking about something that allows you to be interactive mentally, like puzzles. My mom is 89 years old and works 10 Word Search puzzles every day, religiously, except Sundays, when she spends time watching religious channels on television.

I also try to stimulate my mind interactively by doing Crossword puzzles and playing myself on the internet with games such as dominoes and chess. The key is doing something that requires your active participation, not just sitting in front of the television like a vegetable. I have also taken up learning Spanish, with a goal of being fluent within the next two - three years. I don't actually take classes, but I do listen to interactive audio tapes, an hour each day, and encourage others to do the same.The benefit is twofold: Mental

Stimulation and learning a foreign language that I fully intend to use. You are never too old to learn! That's my motto!

Here is a list of **10 stimulating activities Alzheimer patients** recommended by **Advent Health.com - www.adventhealth.com/ blog -**

April 22, 2022:

1. Make a Scrapbook
2. Do Arts and Crafts
3. Play Music
4. Make a Photo Album or Scrapbook
5. Encourage Physical Activity
6. Read the Newspaper
7. Do Puzzles
8. Cook and Bake
9. Keep the Conversation Going
10. Do Chores Together

11

IS THERE A CURE FOR DEMENTIA?

According to the **National Health Service (NHS)** in England, "There is **currently no "cure" for Dementia**. In fact, because **Dementia** is caused by different diseases it is unlikely that there will be a single cure for dementia. Research is aimed at finding cures for **Dementia-causing diseases**, such as **Alzheimer's disease, frontotemporal dementia** and **dementia with Lewy bodies...** "Although a cure may be some years away, there are some very promising advances." – www.nhs.uk page review April 8, 2021

The **Alzheimer Society of Canada** goes on to say, "...These types of **Dementia** are what we call "neurodegenerative". The progression of these **Dementias** cannot be reversed right now; symptoms gradually get worse. But current treatment options and brain-health lifestyle choices can help manage some of the symptoms." - **www.alzheimer.ca - 2023**

12

SOME TIPS FOR LIVING YOUR BEST LIFE WITH DEMENTIA

"A diagnosis of **Dementia** does not mean our life is over. This section provides you with strategies to live well with Dementia, along with tips and advice from other people who are living with **Dementia**." - www.alzheimer.ca - 2023

- Eat as healthy as possible
- If you smoke, try to quit
- If you drink, do so moderately or better yet, quit
- Stay active, socially, as much as possible
- Attempt some form of daily exercise
- Try to stay physically active as best you can
- Try not to stay up late nights, get good rest
- Share what is helping you live well with other Dementia patients

"Stay mentally and socially active. Engaging in mental or social activities **may** help to build up your brain's ability to cope with disease, relieve stress and improve your mood. This means that doing these activities may help to delay, or even prevent, dementia from developing." - www.alzheimers.org.uk - **page review November 25, 2021**

13

I FEEL YOUR PAIN! I TOO SUFFER MEMORY LOSS!

One of the most humbling things in the world is admitting that you have any type of sickness or disease. But, the truth is, if you are willing to do so, you can get the medical or psychiatric help that you need to deal with your Dementia. Also, you will be able to get family members, friends and associates to understand why you behave the way that you do and the frustration you may feel. Understanding is everything!

Personally, I feel the pain of those suffering from Dementia because I have finally come to grips with the fact that I am starting to experience memory loss myself. For too many years, I have ignored the warning signs and that because of my declining memory, I may be a person that may have inherited something that I've witnessed in previous family members.

Up until now, I thought it quite natural to forget key moments and events in my life. But, there are some things that I absolutely should have not forgotten from my past. And, what past that was, something I will save for a future auto-biography! I have definitely lived a full life! I never became a millionaire, but I've had more than a million dollars worth of life experiences! If I were to die tomorrow, I can honestly say that I have lived a life and have had experiences that most people can only dream of.

My life has been anything but boring and I feel that I now have an obligation to give something back for all the blessings that the good Lord has bestowed upon me. The problem is that the events of my life are starting to become sketchy, thus the reason for me to start using the writing skills that I learned during a 20 year career in the U.S. Navy, having retired as a Chief Journalist. I need to use my writing skills to help other people!

I have had too many memorable experiences since graduating from Gary West Side High School in 1973, with a football and track scholarship to South Carolina State College, in Orangeburg, SC. While there, I spent too much time having a good time, partying, cutting classes and chasing women, to graduate with my class.

As a result, I flunked out of school, and made the decision to join the U.S. Navy, where I knew that I would get the discipline that I was lacking going to college so far from home.

Did I turn my life of parting around? Absolutely not! But, going to boot camp, at Great Lakes Naval Station, Waukegan, IL, I was given the opportunity to be placed in a leadership position, since I was a few years older than nearly all of the other members in my camp. I was selected, by my company commander, to the position of Recruit Chief Petty Officer (RPOC) of company 952. I enjoyed leading the 90 plus recruits in my unit and took pride in being in charge of a

"Color Company". We were called the "State Flags" because we wore fancy Navy uniforms, with spats and silver helmets. As an RPOC, I wore Navy Aiguillettes and carried a silver sword, walking alongside my unit, as we carried all 50 state flags and did fancy drilling maneuvers during our graduation ceremony.

After boot camp graduation in 1979, I attended the Defense Informa-tion School (DINFOS), at Fort Benjamin Harrison, Indianapolis, where I attended the Navy School of Journalism. Following graduation, my first Journalist assignment was onboard the pre-commissioning crew of the Navy Auxiliary Oiler, USS Cimarron (AO-177), stationed in San Diego, CA. I don't have to tell you how great it was to be stationed in San Diego! My goodness!

The ship was subsequently assigned to the San Francisco Bay area, where we were berthed at the Naval Supply Center, Oakland, CA, prior to our commissioning ceremony January 10,1981. There I met and married my first wife: Annie Y. Thomas!

In the fall of 1982, the USS Cimarron (AO-177) changed homeports to Pearl Harbor, HI, where we participated in numerous fleet exercises prior to our six-month deployment to the Western Pacific in November 1983. During my deployment, I submitted news articles that were published in the Navy publications: "All Hands Magazine" and "Surface Warfare" magazine. I was also editor/publisher of the USS Cimarron's first "Cruise Book", covering our port visits to: Subic Bay, Republic of the Philippines; Guam; Thailand; Singapore; Pusan Korea and Sasebo, Japan! Following the ship's return home, to Pearl Harbor, my wife, Annie, who was several months pregnant on the date of my departure, gave birth to our son, Thomas on March 19, 1994. After my sea duty tour, I was assigned to the staff of Commander Naval Base, Pearl Harbor, HI.

It was during that period where I went to Chaminade University of Honolulu, using Navy Tuition Assistance, to earn my Bachelors Degree in Criminal Justice, December 8, 1986.

During my four years in Hawaii, the Navy paid for me and my wife to stay in a 15 story high rise apartment, with a sliding glass door, on the patio, down-town, Honolulu, overlooking beautiful Waikiki. We were given the opportunity to enjoy great food, good entertainment, a great night life, and all that the island of Oahu had to offer. When relatives came to visit us, and stayed at our apartment, they weren't in a hurry to go back home! Hawaii was fantastic!

Everything in life is not peaches and cream. My extra-marital adventures would result in a divorce. Totally my fault, followed by being assigned to live in the barracks, on base, prior to my reassignment to the admiral's staff, Naval Station, Treasure Island, CA. Prior to that base closing, I had a great, night view of Alcatraz Island and the skyline of San Francisco.

The rest of my Navy career will be covered in my future autobiography. In it, I will go into more detail of how I was selected to attend the Navy's Officer Candidate School (OCS), attended, partied and flunked out. Of how I was given a second chance and meritorious promoted to Journalist Chief Petty Officer, attended classes nights and weekends, earning my Masters Degree in Public Administration from Troy State University, met my second wife: Olga E. Martinez, who had four kids: Rafaela, Jennifer, Christopher and Michael, while being assigned to the Navy Recruiting Orientation Unit (NORU), Pensacola. FL.

Following the family's move to the San Francisco/Oakland Bay area, I was assigned as the Public Affairs Officer, Navy Recruiting Region West (NAVCRUITAREA 8).

Continuing my philandering ways, I went on to become divorced for my second time. As my step-children will attest, I was a great step-father, but an unfaithful husband. My problem has been that I am liked by everyone who knows me, have a charming personality, get along with everyone who knows me, will give you the shirt off my back in a clutch situation, but have yielded to temptation one time too many when it comes to the opposite sex.

Now, how does the story that I just laid out before you relate to my experiencing the onset of Dementia? Well, for one thing I have trouble remembering names of people that I have just met, can't remember the names of more than a hand-full of my classmates, out of a graduating class or more than 700, can't remember the names of my grade school, junior high school and high school teachers, am always misplacing personal items, need a shopping list if I have to remember more than three items, and I am sure there are other things that I can't remember to include in this list. That is why it is so important for me to document everything, to write down everything, to keep a "To Do List" or "Tickler List" with me at all times. Without which, I struggle to remember! Based on my past, there are some things that I need to forget having done!

Let me say this again for all of those suffering from Dementia or the onset of Dementia, "I feel your pain!" You are not alone!

14

RESOURCES/REFERENCES

World Health Organization (WHO) - 2023:
https://www.who.int/health- topics/dementia#ta b=tab_1

Alzheimer's Association - 2023:
https://www.alz.org/alzheimers-dementia/what-is-dementia

American Seniors Communities (ASC) - February 19, 2015:
https://www.asccare.com/mental-illness-vs-dementia-elderly/#:
~:text=While%20dementia%20does%20affect%20mental,loss
%20and%20trouble%20with%20communicating

Food and Drug Administration (FDA) - News release May 11, 2023:
https://www.fda.gov/news-events/press-announcements/fda-approves-first-drug-treat-agitation-symptoms-associated-dementia-due-alzheimers-disease

Merriam-Webster Dictionary - New release updated May 26, 2026:
https://www.merriam-webster.com/dictionary/dementia#:~:
text=%3A%20a%20usually%20progressive%20condition%20

RESOURCES/REFERENCES

Center for Disease Control and Prevention (CDC) - News release revised April 5, 2019:
https://www.cdc.gov/aging/dementia

National Center for Complementary and Integrative Health (NCCIH) - July 2022:
https://www.nccih.nih.gov/health/tips/things-to-know-about-dietary-supplements-for-cognitive-function-dementia-and-alzheimers-disease

National Health Service England (NHS.uk) - page review April 8, 2021:
https://www.nhs.uk/conditions/dementia/cure

Open Systems Healthcare (OSH) - News release September 6, 2019:
https://opensystemshealthcare.com/knowledge/what-is-dementia-alzheimers

Mayoclinic.org, News release October 12, 2022:
https://www.mayoclinic.org/diseases-conditions/alzheimers-disease/in-depth/alzheimers/art-20048103

Mayoclinic.org, News release April 1, 2023:
https://www.mayoclinic.org/diseases-conditions/primary-progressive-aphasia/symptoms-causes/syc-20350499

Alzheimers.org.uk, News release May 23, 2023:
https://www.alzheimers.org.uk/blog/how-offer-help-someone-dementia-who-doesnt-want-it

Center for Complementary Integrative Health (NCCIH) - News release July 2022:
https://www.nccih.nih.gov/health/providers/digest/dietary-supplements-and-cognitive-function-dementia-and-alzheimers-disease

Better Health Channel - May 31, 2014:
https://www.betterhealth.vic.gov.au/health/conditionsand treatments/dementia-early-signs

Mayoclinic.org - News release October 12, 2022:
https://www.mayoclinic.org/diseases-conditions/alzheimers-disease/in-depth/alzheimers/art-20048103

Alzheimers.org.uk, News release February 21, 2022:
https://www.alzheimers.org.uk/blog/difference-between-dementia-alzheimers-disease#:~:text=Alzheimer's%20disease%20s tarts%20 in%20the,to%20be%20called%20'dementia

Food and Drug Administration (FDA) - News release October 26, 2022
https://www.fda.gov/food/information-consumers-using-dietary-supplements/questions-and-answers-dietary-supplemen ts#: ~:text=However%2C%20by%20law%2C%20FDA%20does,(e.g.% 2C%20health%20claims)

Adventhealth.com/blog - News release April 22, 2022:
https://www.adventhealth.com/blog/10-stimulating-activities-alzheimers-disease-patients

RESOURCES/REFERENCES

CBS News - May 24, 2023:
www.cbsnews.com
https://www.cbsnews.com/boston/news/brigham-and-womens-study-daily-multivitamin-improve-brain-function-older-adults/#:~:text=BOSTON%20%2D%20Taking%20a%20daily%20 multivitamin,over%20a%20three%2Dyear%20period

Careforth.com, article by Angela Stringfellow, May 17, 2018:
https://www.careforth.com/blog/what-are-the-best-vitamins-for-dementia-patients-11-vitamins-minerals-and-herbs-to-improve-well-being

Harvard Healthcare - August 12, 2022:
https://www.health.harvard.edu/topics/memory#:~:text= Regular%20exercise%20boosts%20the%20growth,to%20nine% 20ho urs%20each%20night

Alzheimer's Association:
https://www.alz.org/professionals/professional-providers/dementia_ care_practice_recommendations

Alzheimer[s Association:
https://www.alz.org/alzheimers-dementia/treatments/ alternative-treatments

Medical NewsToday, News release June 30, 2022:
www.medical-newstoday
https://www.medicalnewstoday.com/articles/dementia-and-anger -at-loved-ones

Healthline.com, Medical review February 14, 2022:
https://www.healthline.com/health/dementia

Food and Drug Administration (FDA), Review June 2, 2022:
https://www.fda.gov/consumers/consumer-updates/fda-101-dietary-supplements

Alzheimer Society of Canada - 2023:
https://alzheimer.ca/en/help-support/im-caring-person-living-dementia/what-expect-persons-dementia-progresses#:~:text=There%20is%20currently%20no%20cure,now%3B%20symptoms%20gradually%20get%20worse

Alzheimer's Society - United Kingdom, page review November 25, 2021
https://www.alzheimers.org.uk/about-dementia/risk-factors-and-prevention/how-reduce-your-risk-alzheimers-and-other-dementias#:~:text=5.-,Stay%20mentally%20and%20socially%20active,even%20prevent%2C%20dementia%20from%20developing

15

CONCLUSION

Writing this book was a real learning experience for me! I did not know that **Dementia** was an **umbrella term** for different memory loss ailments. I always thought that **Alzheimer's disease** and **Dementia** were one and the same. I have become aware of the frustration and anguish that it causes victims as well as family, friends and associates. I pray that modern science can come up with a definite cure to prevent this from happening to future generations.

My heart goes out to those who have **Alzheimer's**, **Dementia**, and other mental problems that rob people of cherished experiences each of us deserves to have in our memory banks until we die. It is sort of like having all of your family photo albums burn up in a fire, depriving you of photos of your loved-ones and friends, and the experiences associated with each photo. People who have had photos albums destroyed, or photos lost, understand the power of a photo or a song to remind us of enjoyable experiences. Think about how you would feel if all your photo albums, baby pictures, etc. were destroyed! That's almost what it feels like to lose your memory!

The human mind is much like a camera and records mental photos and images of the past. **Altzheimer's**, **Dementia** and its related illnesses, serve to delete those mental images, leading to frustration and anguish!

There is not one of us who does not know of someone, whether family, friend or neighbor, who has not experienced or witnessed someone suffering from **Dementia** or some form of memory loss! We have the responsibility to show them that we care, so that they can have the best quality of life possible for the remainder of their lives.

I sincerely hope that this book has been informative and useful to those who read it and humbly ask that you give an honest review of the book, which will allow me to improve on the next one. If you enjoy this one, **email me** to let me know your thoughts and what improvements you'd like to see Volume 2.

May the Lord continue to bless each and every one of you as well as your family members! Be blessed!

—**Warren A. Patton**
wapatton@earthlink.net

www.ingramcontent.com/pod-product-compliance
Lightning Source LLC
LaVergne TN
LVHW041555070526
838199LV00046B/1986